REIKI: THE DEFINITIVE BEGINNER'S GUIDE

Learn the Healing Powers of Reiki to Achieve
Peace of Mind & Re-Energize your Life!

by Dominique Atkinson

© 2017 by Dominique Atkinson
© 2017 by ALEX-PUBLISHING

Published by:

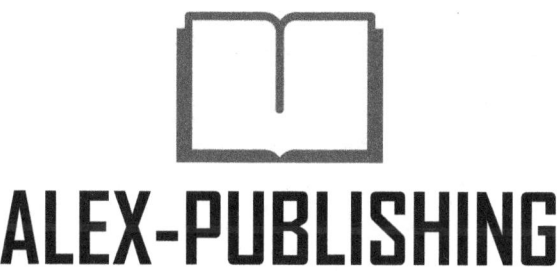

ALEX-PUBLISHING

DISCLAIMER

Note from the Author:

Welcome to the amazing world of Reiki! As many of you know from some of my other books, this has been a passion of mine for many years. I'm blessed to have had incredible teacher's that have guided me in my practice, and I'm thrilled that you will allow me to help you learn this beautiful and ancient philosophy and way of life. The final objective is to achieve better health, a calmer mind and a more peaceful spirit.

Ever since I was a child, I've always taken the road less travelled. To me, the world was magical. As I got older, my peers grew more cynical and pragmatic, but I never lost that vital curiosity. I still saw the nature of the universe as a vast sea of possibilities and puzzles to solve. I wanted to understand things in a way that nobody understood before. I wanted to change things and positively affect other people. When I was a teenager my curiosities lead me down a different path. I started studying different religions and different ancient philosophies.

Early on, I became interest in Reiki. The idea that there was a way to harness the fundamental power of the universe intrigued me, and using it to heal others; in body, mind and spirit. Reiki is divided into different levels. The first Reiki level can be taught in the course of a weekend but takes years of patient study and practice to become a Reiki Master Teacher.

Reiki will change your life. By learning it, you will also have the tools to change the lives of others, and there's nothing more beautiful than compassionate love and healing.

Let's get started!!

Best,

Dominique Atkinson

TABLE OF CONTENTS

Introduction

Imagine you are standing in a powerful storm. The wind is blowing through your hair, the trees are swaying violently. Lightning strikes and you jump. You can feel that palpable electric tension flowing through you and see it everywhere around you. Your skin tingles, your heart rushes and you know, somehow, that something is there.

Everything is made up of energy. Einstein's fundamental discovery was the idea that everything material takes its source from energy. That fundamental principle is represented in his famous equation, $E = mc^2$. Cultures around the world, from the ancient Greeks to the Japanese have always talked about the energetic nature of the universe. They have known well before modern scientists that the world is fundamentally composed of a life force that makes up everything.

That energy is powerful and dynamic. It's the very essence of life present in all things. It is that surging power flowing through the storm. It is that rush of adrenaline you get. It's that healing touch of a mother or a lover. It's that tenderness you feel inside and that love you give to another person. It can heal us, change us and shape us because it's the power that flows through all of us.

Einstein said that rather than being made of palpable materials, all matter is composed of small vortices of energy. Everyone knows what happened with Einstein's theories. By understanding the fundamental nature of the universe, man was able to create the most powerful destructive force in existence. The power of energy is the power of the universe. It can do great things. It can destroy mountains, topple empires, bring a man from rags to riches, and it can heal. The question is how do you harness it for good? How do you use it to influence your life? How do you use it to heal yourself and others?

Harnessing the power of energy is the most powerful tool a man has. By unlocking the power of the universe, he can reach his fullest potential and move past any obstacle it has. This power is a part of everything, so it can influence everything.

In this book, you will learn to harness this power, not for destructive means, but for the ability to heal yourself and others. Healing is the most powerful blessing we can give to one another. When we heal others, we are also healing ourselves and creating a better world. By learning to harness this energy to help others, we can learn to better ourselves and the lives of other people. Healing somebody is the most powerful gift we can give.

Chapter 1 – What is Reiki?

"It is much better to give this power widely to a lot of people in the world and enjoy it among them than to keep it exclusively," - Usui-Sensei Founder of the Reiki System

Some say it was in 1914, others say it was 1922. Either way, it was a fateful year. A young Buddhist priest, who had traveled the world, and learned many things fasted on Mt. Kurama for 21 days. He sat in silent contemplation, starving and weak from the hunger. His journey was a spiritual one, one of inner sacrifice for a higher goal.

He came to what is called a Kami tree, a place where rest and peace are found. On the 21st day, he felt something. He sensed the energy of everything flowing through him. He sensed the power of nature and the world. He was attuned to the life-force.

Usui-Sensei came from a spiritual tradition of service. He believed in the idea that one should give up the ego because it blocks us from helping others. When we give up selfish desires, we break down the barriers to compassion and love.

Reiki reflects that spirit of service and so does Mikao Usui. He didn't just want to heal people, but heal others. It's about teaching others to fish and helping them heal others in the spirit of service.

Where Does the Word Come From?

Reiki's etymology is a fantastic symbol for explaining the system. It's a Japanese word that is broken up into two parts with separate meanings. Rei is God's wisdom or higher power. It's his light that shines down on us when we are happy or feeling excited. It's the light of the sun, the awe inspiring vision of the stars. That feeling we get when we see those things that is Rei. Ki is the life-force that flows through everything. It's the power of the wind, that which moves everything and that which is the catalyst for change.

By putting these things together we get Reiki. That means that Reiki is taking the spiritual power of God and using it to direct the power of Ki. By spiritually directing energy, you give it a life of its own. Consider that power of the Universe a dormant force, waiting to be directed. Reiki imbues that power with love and light and channels it into a palpable force.

The Reiki Practice

When a person gets hurt, there is a universal reaction to that stimuli. When you have a headache, you cradle your head or massage your temples. When a child comes up to his mother to show her a cut, she kisses it. If you hit your leg, you rub it. There's something about touch that heals people.

Maybe it's the contact that we feel. It's the desire to reach out to another person when we are hurt. It's the pain of being unloved. It's the reassurance and the love that people need. Pain isn't just a physical thing. There is a union between our minds, our souls, and our bodies. That union needs to be treated fully.

The power of touch is the essential Reiki practice. It's about utilizing Ki and channeling it through your hands to provide the love and the light people need to heal. We all do this naturally, by instinct. We all feel the need to reach out to others when we are in pain. We need that touch to satisfy something inside of us.

Reiki can be as simple as rubbing somebody's shoulder or shaking their hands. The slightest touch can change lives and by channeling the power of Reiki we can heal others in ways that we never thought possible.

Practitioners of Reiki hone their craft by learning first to feel the power that resides in all things and then by learning to utilize it. They learn points throughout the body that need to be healed. They learn to direct that power through an individual to heal them. They learn to feel out the points in the body that are tied up and need to be healed. They learn how to massage away worries and pains. They learn how to soothe the soul and ease the mind.

The System

Reiki is divided into different schools. The original school was started by Usui-Sensei in the 1920s since then the practice has branched off into hundreds of schools and travelled to the west.

Every school has its own system of learning and teaching individuals to use the practice, but there is a standard format. Normally, a person is taught in levels or degrees of initiation which they receive through master teachers. There are usually three levels of mastery which begin from level one to level three. After that, a person is taught to become a master teacher by apprenticing with another master teacher.

Each level is not passed onto the student through traditional methods. Instead, it is taught to them through the use of attunement. This is the practice of handing over a Reiki symbol to another student. By doing so, the power of Reiki is transferred to them.

Undertaking the process of learning Reiki is a serious thing. Reiki is not just about healing others, it's about teaching others how to heal. By doing so, master teachers are embarking on a journey of compassion and service. Healing others and teaching them to heal others is sacred.

Chapter 2 – The Benefits of Reiki

Your body is more than just a collection of cells, organs, and tissues. There is an essence that binds all of your working parts together and makes you the person you are. In terms of Reiki healing that invisible element that the body is balanced by is the life force energy, Ki. Imbalances in the energy and blockages to its flow can result from any number of negative physical and emotional feelings, whether it be an injury, an illness, or destructive emotions such as anger, fear, or self-depreciation and lack of esteem.

While Reiki should not be used as an alternative to seeking medical attention at times of need, the gentle energy working of Reiki healing on the body means that imbalances in Ki can be restored. Once the natural flow of life force energy is restored, continued Reiki sessions can ensure it is maintained. Excellent results are seen when Reiki is used to treat and heal any number of emotional, physical, or spiritual issues resulting in a reduction of pain, symptoms, and an overall sense of comfort.

Stress reduction and relaxation are a key benefit to the practice of Reiki and many of the health benefits can be attributed to the body's response to a stress free and relaxed state being enabled. This improves our body's natural defenses, healing abilities, and improves general health and well-being. By gently balancing the Ki, the natural remedy Reiki, will leave you feeling healthier, more contented, and less stressed.

Our body's natural abilities to heal and recover are improved when we are relaxed and free from stress. When in physical pain or experiencing emotional distresses our body produces hormones which benefit us in the short term. The production of stress hormones allow us to react to whatever it is causing us stress, it is commonly termed a fight or flight state and results. When faced with an immediate crisis we can react better due to the stimulus that stress hormones such as noradrenaline produce, however, over longer periods of time these hormones build up and the effect on the body becomes toxic. Using Reiki to relax and reduce the physical impact of stresses on our health causes a reduction in the hormones produced, allowing the patient to cope better with anxieties and to deal more successfully with physical pain.

Reiki healing can be utilized to concentrate solely on a problem area such as a localized injury or symptoms of a disease or illness that affect only one or two areas of the body. As Ki flows through the entire body, one of the favored practices within Reiki is to take a whole body approach. Working not only to alleviate certain symptoms but to restore the balances of energies through the entire body. This can benefit us in a number of ways, allowing a faster recovery from illness or injury or alleviating the symptoms of more chronic diseases. Once a level of recovery has been achieved continued whole body Reiki healing can bring about a sustainable change in your state of consciousness enabling you to maintain a sense of contentment and an internal seat of subtle confidence protecting and defending you from succumbing to further anxiety caused by environmental stressors. Not only can Reiki help you recover, but it can also help you achieve a state of body and mind where you are better able to deal with what life has to throw at you.

When we are in good health, we have the capacity to regain our natural healing ability. Daily practice of Reiki will endure good health of the body. It will rid the body of stressors, toxins, anxiety and depression by opening up the energy reservoirs. When a person has good and sustainable health, your body's natural defences will always be up. This will create balance in the body which will mean that your health is in order. Then as a result that person will gain a better perspective on life. Reiki can also provide extra energy when most at need, in times of illness.

Reiki healing methods aggregates Western and Eastern medicine, so everyone can benefit from it. As well as being useful to humans, it is also very beneficial to animals and plants. Reiki healing energy provides quick pain relief and instant comfort.

Examples of how Reiki Healing can Improve your Health

Reiki can help you by creating a deep state of relaxation which aids the body by reducing tension and releasing stresses. This has the beneficial effect of reducing the blood pressure and the deep relaxing state can improve the quality of sleep you get further allowing the body a chance to recover and to recuperate, whether that be an accumulation of stress or general aches and pains from day to day living, or, more specific issues arising from injury, chronic disease, or mental illness.

Reiki can be used to focus the body's natural healing energies to acute injuries or chronic causes of pain, reducing pain. Reiki masters have even used the life force energies to induce such deep states of relaxation that it has circumvented the need for heavy anesthesia during invasive surgical procedures. Reiki is often utilized in order to speed up the recovery period following surgical anesthesia and despite being around as a Japanese practice since 1922 it is now becoming more and more recognized as an alternative and complementary therapy in Western medical circles.

Reiki is also increasingly being used to counteract the imbalances of the body caused by some drugs. Not only is this anesthetic drugs and long term pain relievers, but Reiki can reduce the harmful side effects of drugs such as chemotherapy treatments.

Reiki healing has recognized effects on a person's emotional well-being. This is achieved by balancing the life force, and removing a build-up of toxins, thus allowing the endocrine system to reach an equilibrium state, bringing the body into a state of harmony and balance. Reiki healing can be used to deal with acute anxiety disorders as well as chronic disorders such as depression. Reiki can also be beneficial in the breaking of addiction.

By enabling the body to achieve and maintain a balance Reiki supports the natural immune system enabling the recipient to successfully defend against viral and bacterial illnesses. This increase in protection can also be witnessed as a sense of increased vitality and feelings of youthfulness and well-being prolonging the aging process and giving a 'new lease of life'.

The natural balancing of Reiki healing is often utilized by practitioners to reinforce the benefits of other therapies such as homeopathic, massage, and aromatherapy. When used to complement other alternative therapies as well as traditional medicine the benefits of combined therapies are more sustainable as the non-invasive nature of Reiki healing enables it to be utilized across a wide range of patients, including the non-human kind as Reiki can also be used to improve the well-being of animals and is becoming more popular as a treatment for pets suffering from medical conditions or behavioral issues. While the most intense Reiki healing will be performed by a registered practicing Reiki Master, healing energies can be used at any moment, at any time, and on anybody.

Chapter 3 - Reiki Symbol Meanings

More practiced Reiki healers who have attained the second or Master level of Reiki are able to use the symbols sacred to Reiki. When using Reiki symbols the healer brings the person to be healed into the same zone of Ki, so the healer and the recipient are attuned to each other. This enables the healing energy of the practitioner to interact with that of their subject so the healer can be guided by intuition rather than simply carrying out a step by step generalized Reiki massage. When used during healing sessions they provide both protection and healing to the subject. The Reiki healer will use the symbols in order to focus their attention to connect with different levels of Ki using the appropriate symbol in order to activate and boost their Reiki energy. Reiki symbols have been passed down from Master to Master.

When performing a Reiki healing the symbols have to be activated. This can be done in various different ways. The vital part of the successful use of Reiki symbols comes from the Reiki healer and the belief that the symbol can be used within healing and the intention. The symbols should then be applied initially on the healer's hands and then drawn or visualized on the crown chakra, the hands of the subject, and on any particular area that needs to be treated.

When initially introducing Reiki symbols into your healing sessions you can bring them into the healing realm of Ki by spelling out the name of the symbol three times, tracing the shape with your finger, using the palm of your hand to draw the symbol light on or above the person you are healing, drawing them through visualization through your third eye, or by simply visualizing and concentrating on the shape of the symbol. The most important aspect of using the symbols is that you intend for the symbol to assist you and draw on the associated energy during your Reiki healing. Masters of Reiki healing are so practiced in the use of the symbols that the physical aspect of the symbol becomes unnecessary and the intention and focus of the energies associated with each symbol becomes the center of their energy balancing.

There are five traditional symbols of Reiki. Each has a different purpose and can be used in different manners to accentuate and focus the healing powers of Reiki. They were originally introduced by the Japanese monk Usui in order to assist students of Reiki in focusing their intent and to attune their Ki with their subjects.

The most powerful of all the Reiki symbols is the Master Symbol: Dai Ko Myo. Dai Ko Myo is used to bring healing to the soul and when utilized correctly can bring about life changes for the Reiki healer and the subject. It deals with the root causes of disease and illness by providing peace and enlightenment and aligning the soul and the spiritual self. The effect of Dai Ko Myo is to enable the subject to become more psychically attuned and intuitive to their own needs.

The Power Symbol: Cho Ku Ray is primarily used in order to raise the level of Reiki power. It means I have the key. It enables the healer to draw energy from the environment and focus it where the healer intends. Again it is the intention of the healer to draw that power and focus it that gives Cho Ku Ray its power. When using Cho Ku Ray the words can be silently thought three times or the symbol can be traced over the healer or the subject.

Cho Ku Ray is a versatile symbol and can be used to manifest healing energies, to cleanse the spiritual body from negative energy – this can be both within the Ki of the subject, or in an area such as a hospital or an area where an accident or injury has occurred. Cho Ku Ray can also be used to cleanse herbal poultices, medical drugs, food, and water.

This symbol is often used in order to increase the healing power of other Reiki symbols and to ensure that energies that have been raised during healing treatments are protected and maintained. Cho Ku Ray is also excellent when focusing healing powers on specific areas of the body. If you want to use the Cho Ku Ray symbol on yourself then you should focus on the mirror image, reversing it, and that will channel the increased energies inward rather than outward.

The symbol used primarily in order to deal with emotional healing and providing a sense of calm to the recipient of healing is the Mental / Emotional symbol Sei Hei Ki. Sei Hei Ki means the key of the universe. This symbol provides emotional cleansing and psychic protection. When dealing with afflictions that are governed by the mind as well as the body such as addiction, post-traumatic stress, and anxiety the symbol Sei Hei Ki is brought into play. A Reiki healer will use Sei Hei Ki when performing meditations prior to a healing session in order to cleanse their own Ki and make them more receptive and intuitive in their healing of another. The Mental / Emotional symbol provides balance and harmony by clearing emotional blockages, removing bad vibrations, and eliminating negative energies.

Reiki healing can be carried out both within close proximity where the healer will place their hands either above or lightly on their subject, or, remotely across distance. Healing can be carried out by focusing the life energies and sending Reiki across time and distance. Reiki healing can be transported to anyone and anything at any time utilizing the Distance Symbol: Hon Sha Ze Sho Nen. Due to the shape of the symbol this can also be referred to as the pagoda symbol.

One of the main purposes of Reiki healing is to balance the life energies in the healer and in the subject. It is the unblocking and balancing of Ki that provides an access to the other aspects of Reiki. The freedom of energy flow within the spirit allows Reiki to benefit the whole body. The symbol used for balancing and grounding Ki and unblocking energy chakras to allow the flow of healing spiritual energy through the body is Tam-A-Ra-Sha or the Balancing Factor. If Tam-A-Ra-Sha is focused on a point of pain it can be used by a healer to reduce or remove that pain.

Whichever of the Reiki symbols you are using in your healing of another or of yourself the most important aspect is that the symbols are activated and that the focus is in the intention of performing the action of the symbol itself. Reiki symbols provide access to specific healing energies, used in combination they are a powerful tool to the healer and a source of positive healing for the recipient. When first working with Reiki symbols it might be difficult to remember the Reiki names for each of the symbols, using the alternative name for the symbol will not have any detriment to the symbol's use providing the intention is as strong, for example, if you're unable to remember Cho Ku Ray during a healing session it is possible to substitute the Reiki name with its alias: The Power Symbol.

Chapter 4 – The Three Pillars of Reiki

The energies of Reiki are always present and flowing. Reiki healing can be spontaneous and drawing on the energy can be immediate, however, as already seen when utilizing Reiki symbols it is the intention of a healer to use Reiki to promote well-being and influence the spiritual healing energy of themselves or a recipient that gives Reiki a focused power. For this reason it is important that a practitioner of Reiki healing prepare themselves prior to undertaking Reiki healing.

Dr Usui proposed and taught that there were three stages that promote the influences of Reiki and that these should be undertaken prior to using Reiki. These three stages enhance the effect that a Reiki healing session has by enabling the healer to draw upon more energy, focus more clearly, and to attune themselves to Ki and the intention to heal. The three stages of Reiki are termed the three pillars.

The three pillars of Reiki are used to empower Reiki sessions. By performing the three pillars prior to undertaking a healing session you introduce a clear intention into the healing. Throughout any life experience we are aware that anything conducted with a powerful intention will achieve better results than anything undertaken unintentionally or without a focus drawn through preparation.

The first of the three pillars is termed Gassho and is performed by the Reiki healer prior to the healing session. It is used to provide calm and focus within the healer and to allow the healing energy to flow within them. The healer centers themselves by following a simple meditation. The term Gassho means two hands coming together.

In order to perform Gassho you must place your hands together, fingertips touching, in a prayer position in front of the heart. When placing the hands together you connect the energy meridians that end in the hands creating a circular flow of energy through your body. You should concentrate on this flow of energy and give thanks for Reiki, for the presence of others, and for the intended recipient of your Reiki healing. You need to focus on the sensations of your hands touching, the heat and light pressure within your fingertips. You need to try to relax, clear your mind, and focus only on the energy within you. When aware of the energy and relaxed within the meditation you must ask for the energy to flow within you and through you mentally voicing the intention to use the healing energy of Reiki.

The second pillar of Reiki healing is the indication of the Reiki Power or Reiji-Ho. Reiki power is indicated by the word Reiji, and the word Ho relates to the method in which Reiki power is used. You don't have to talk out loud to perform any of the pillars of Reiki, but in this second pillar you are repeating the request within Gassho for the energy of Reiki to flow through you, you are also asking for the energy to be used for healing, and that you will be guided in allowing the energy to flow where it is needed.

Reiji-Ho is performed by interlacing the fingers and crossing the thumbs in front of the heart. You must make a connection with the energy of Reiki and again ask for the energies to flow through you. This request should be made three times. Once you have done this you must ask that the Reiki power can be used by you to heal. You must state your intention, ask for protection, and ask for the Reiki powers to be used ethically and cleanly.

There is a final stage to Reiji-Ho before you can move on to healing. This is to ask for the energies to be guided to the correct places. In order to do this you need to bring your hands up to the third eye. During the second stage you have aligned your intention to heal with the good for your recipient. The third stage is carried out to ensure that the energies are used where they are needed. You're asking for Reiki to guide your energy and to soothe, heal, and repair the recipient. You need to trust that Reiki will guide your healing energies and that even if you're not aware of where the energy is needed, that by following the second pillar that Reiki spirit guides will ensure that the maximum good of the recipient is matched with your deepest intention to heal.

The third pillar of Reiki is the treatment, or Chiryo. This is performed to create a connection between you and your recipient. Following the completion of Gassho and Reihi-Ho you have centered yourself and given thanks for Reiki spiritual healing, you have asked that Reiki flow through you, and you have stated your intention to use your Reiki energies for the good of your recipient. By placing the palm of your dominant hand to the crown chakra of the recipient you now bind yourself to them, allowing your energies to merge with theirs and flow around their body.

You must hold your hand to their crown chakra until you feel the energies flowing between their crown chakra and your hand. You may feel this in the form or a heat or a tingling energy. This is feedback of the Reiki energy flowing from your hand, through their body, and back again. This can also be termed hibiki. When experiencing hibiki there is often a sense of inspiration or an impulse to move the hand to another area of the recipient's body, this is the Reiki spirit guides leading you to the areas that require healing.

Reiki healing can be performed without first embracing the three pillars of Reiki, however, the powerful intention gained by first preparing and centering yourself in order to heal using Reiki spiritual energy will significantly enhance the effects of any Reiki healing session. Respecting the traditions of Reiki and performing the three pillars prior to any treatment will increase the power of your Reiki and the benefits your recipient gains from their healing session.

Chapter 5 – Spiritual Healing Energy

Reiki and spiritual healing should not be mistaken for a religious practice. There are no religious aspects to the healing energies associated with Reiki. Within the realm of Reiki energy it does not matter whether you are a religious person or not, and if you are it does not matter which religion you subscribe to. No matter what religion, race, or sex you are Reiki energy is available to you. All you need is to acknowledge that the energy of Reiki is open to you, to give thanks for that energy, ask for the energy to be made available to you, and to share your intention for its use for the benefit of another.

In order to consider spiritual healing energy we first need to take a look at what is meant by the term spiritual healing. The term spiritual healing conjures different impressions depending on the perspective of the person examining the phenomenon. A priest may consider that spiritual healing comes directly from God, or from Jesus Christ. There are in fact some students of Reiki who believe that Jesus may have been one of the first practitioners of Reiki healing. A scientist who studies spiritual healing may be searching for tangible evidence such as changes in measured brain waves or in tested blood chemicals. For some the idea of spiritual healing is linked to faith that the healing process will provide them comfort and improve their well-being.

The main idea of spiritual healing is that it encompasses the whole being. Unlike medicine which may focus solely on a particular ailment, spiritual healing is a holistic process, improving general health and state of mind as well as focusing on particular illnesses or injuries. By healing the whole mind, body, and spirit rather than only one aspect you not only improve the condition, but you're also better able to deal with any chronic ailments.

There are some schools of thought that now suggest that the term spiritual healing should be replaced by the term energy healing due to the differing connotations that the term spiritual has amongst different groups of people. The term energy healing does not have as many interpretations, different people may believe that the source of the energy varies. While some may attribute the energy to a God others may understand it to come from the nature of the universe.

There is nothing supernatural about healing energies. Everything in the universe is made up of energy. It is the way in which these energies vibrate together that differentiate between what would generally be considered to be living and non-living, but something as inanimate as a rock still has energy and energy vibrations. They are just slower. There are various different names for the life-force which inhabits humans, it is perhaps most commonly termed the soul or the spirit.

Connecting with this life force or soul is how spiritual healers such as Reiki practitioners are able to heal. Connection and healing is guided by Reiki Guides. Not all Reiki healers will be aware of the presence of their guides, but others may be very aware of their presence and the guidance that is offered to them during healing sessions. Different practitioners may feel their guidance in different ways, they may see images of parts of the body or mind that need attention, or they may feel like their hands are moving automatically over the body of the recipient without conscious intent. The guide assists the healer by ensuring they are able to connect with new levels of energy and adjust to these changes while carrying out healing sessions.

The interaction a healer has with their guide varies. The communication between a healer and their guide(s) takes time and practice. Be assured however, that if you begin to practice Reiki that you will have some connection with your Reiki guides. You may also feel the presence of others while treating. The guides of other healers may come to assist, especially if a healer utilizes the Hon Sha Ze Sho Nen symbol for distance healing. In addition it is believed by many that the spirit guides of the recipient may also assist in guiding the Reiki energy to the appropriate areas within their mind, body, and soul in order for them to gain maximum benefit and protection from the Reiki energies.

If you are new to performing Reiki you may not be aware of the presence of a Reiki Guide. If you need the assistance of your guide then all you have to do is ask them, and then be patient in learning how to interpret their answer. It may not be immediately clear, but if you try too hard to understand it will become more difficult. The relationship between a healer and their spirit guide is instinctive and natural and cannot be forced.

Not everyone is comfortable with the notion of spirit guides and Reiki guides. The power of Reiki will not be adversely affected by electing not to communicate with your Reiki guide. Your healing ability will be as strong, providing that you ensure that you undertake the three pillars of Reiki prior to a treatment and that you activate and utilize the most appropriate symbols to focus and communicate your intent.

Chapter 6 – Techniques

Reiki techniques are employed for specific purposes dependent on the requirements of the individual. Techniques have evolved significantly over time. Originally Reiki techniques were very advanced and were only taught by Usui-Sensei to select Reiki masters of the day. In more recent times Reiki techniques have been developed to become more accessible so that all practitioners of Reiki may be able to avail of these techniques. Below are some of the most common techniques used in Reiki today.

Gassho, as previously discussed, is a meditation technique that consists of the fingers being pressed lightly together in front of the chest, normally without touching the chest. Gassho is the first pillar and one of the core techniques used in Reiki and features regularly in all Reiki technique. Gassho is vitally important and is used to relax and to focus the Reiki practitioner before or after other Reiki techniques.

Kenyoku-ho, also known as dry bathing is a technique used to cleanse the practitioner's energies. This is normally carried out before and after treatment. It can also be employed to disconnect us from the physical world or from others. To carry out Kenyoku-ho, place a palm on the opposite shoulder and gently brush the bad energy down and away from the torso. As you brush, breathe out all bad energy with a quiet 'ha' sound. Repeat this process on the opposite side of your body. Kenyoku-ho is then repeated starting from the shoulder and cleansing and brushing the arms in the same way. Kenyoku-ho should be carried out as many times as necessary until the practitioner feels cleansed.

Chiryo is a method of detoxification and the passing of energy from one individual or area to another. There are several forms of Chiryo such as Enkaku Chiryo (Using Chiryu over long distances) and Heso Chiryo-ho (Chiryo in which the practitioner uses the navel or stomach area more centrally in treatment. This technique is often carried out to help with balance and posture. A typical way of performing Chiryo is for the practitioners to stand side by side, and for the Reiki master to physically touch the client in significant areas for example at the temples (crown chakra) or the small of the back (base chakra).

Koki-ho is the breathing technique employed by teachers to breathe out negative energy and breathe in positive energy. This technique is also regularly used for different types of treatments and throughout the practice of Reiki in general.

A slightly more advanced breathing technique than Koki-ho is Joshin Koki-ho which means upper-body breathing. For Joshin Koki-ho it is best to start in a neutral seated position using Gassho to calm the mind. The use of different hand positions is common, such as palms facing to the sky and hands resting palm up in the practitioner's lap. On the in-breath, the practitioner should feel and imagine Reiki gathering in their mind then, subsequently on the out breath, feel the Reiki disperse to the space in which Joshin Koki-ho is being carried out.

One of the most important Reiki techniques is Hatsurei-ho. It is known by all Reiki practitioners to be one of the key aspects of Reiki and was what Dr. Usui considered to be most meaningful in all Reiki practice, it is said. Hasurei-ho is used to build energy and self-empowerment. It is a combination of all the meditation techniques already discussed. The practitioner should cleanse using Kenyoku-ho before starting. It involves being seated in a Seishin Touitsu position (the standard, neutral Reiki position) and focusing on the Reiki energy using the Gassho and Koki-ho techniques. The Reiki light is breathed in and contained in the self and then breathed out to the surrounding space, ensuring that energy is contained within as well.

The technique commonly used by Reiki masters and practitioners when working with clients who require healing is called Byosen Reikan-ho. It is also referred to as scanning, especially in western cultures. It is the Reiki method of diagnosis. It can be used to determine physical as well as psychological ailments. After appropriate preparation, the practitioner passes their hands over the client's body. Some people physically touch for this method, others pass their hands over the body without actually touching it. It should be noted that scanning should be holistic; that is to say a complete examination of the body, not just focused on areas where the client claims to be in pain. This is because the problem area in a client might be completely different to where the client actually feels pain. The practitioner should feel types of energy in their hands as they pass over the problem area. Examples of different types of energy might be pulsating or buzzing. Different types of energy and feeling represent different issues e.g. attraction to the area generally means that attention is needed in that area.

Nentatsu-ho is the technique used by Reiki practitioners to transform negative energy, habits and feelings into positive ones. This is generally achieved with the use of symbols as opposed to breathing as is the case with Koki-ho. With the aid of symbols an affirmation is meditated upon. The practitioner imagines the negative energy or issue to have been transformed into something positive. The affirmation is thought of in the past, as if the problem has already been resolved. The affirmation is generally meditated upon for five minutes.

Other common techniques include Raiji-ho (which is the practice of calling guides) as well as Reiki Mawashi (Raiki carried out in a circle by several practitioners) and Shu Chu Reiki (The concentration of energy into one area. This generally occurs when a member of a party needs healing or help and other practitioners focus their energies toward the individual to aid in their recovery.

Reiki practitioners should always prepare spiritually for their techniques and feel emotionally and spiritually ready before carrying out Reiki techniques. There should be a very distinct change in the aura of the individual during the time techniques are being carried out. There always must be a clear distinction in the mind between normal life and Reiki practice. Practitioners usually distinguish from the normal and the spiritual by physically stating when they begin for example 'I am now beginning Natatsu-ho.'

Chapter 7 – 10 Massage Ideas for Beginners

The following is set of ideas that anybody who wants to practice Reiki treatment can think about and employ. These are not a set of strict guidelines but rather ideas that have been shown to work by Reiki practitioners and masters through the ages. The purpose of a Reiki massage is to release stress, to discover and resolve problem areas in a person, to heal (both physically and spiritually) and to treat, unblock and examine the energy in a person.

Firstly to clarify; a Reiki energy massage is not the same as a traditional massage that everybody is familiar with. With traditional massage therapy, muscle groups are physically manipulated and maneuvered in order to release physical tension that the client may have. In comparison to this, a Reiki massage is non-invasive. The client remains fully clothed. There are no oils involved. Indeed, a Reiki massage may be carried out without any physical touching at all, although this is less common.

The second idea to think about when performing a Reiki massage is the use of music. The introduction of appropriate music into Reiki therapy sessions has proven to have an extremely relaxing quality on both practitioners and clients. The music should be calming, soothing and be completely unobtrusive to the session. The hope is that a lovely, relaxing, background atmosphere will be created. Most Reiki practitioners of today would use music as a tool during massage treatments. Music for Reiki is freely available on the internet for anybody to avail of. This idea of using music in sessions stretches all the way back to the foundation of Reiki. Dr. Usui would prepare for treatment with a song. Many Reiki practitioners chant or hum or even recite some simple lines of traditional poetry to focus and relax the mind and spirit before and during treatment.

The chakras are a very useful guide for practitioners when carrying out Reiki massage therapy. Chakras are the energy centers in living entities. In Reiki there are seven chakras. The goal is to help energy to flow though the chakra areas. Energy blockages in the chakras are what generally lead to problems that the client might be experiencing. The seven chakras are responsible for different areas of our life. The following is a brief summary of the seven chakras. The chakras are represented by the seven colors red, orange, yellow, green, blue, indigo and violet (from base to crown). They spread from the crown chakra at the top of the head down to the root chakra at the base of the spine. Having a good knowledge of the chakras works as a strong foundation for administering successful Reiki massage therapy.

The fourth idea to consider when discussing Reiki energy massage therapy is the idea of holistic treatment. Each area of the body should be examined in turn from the head to the toes. It is useful as a practitioner to consider each body part in turn. After necessary preparation, one might start with the head of the client. Here the practitioner focuses on resolving any energy issues, pinpointing potential problems, reinforcing positive energy and withdrawing negative energy from this area of the body. After any issues in this area have been resolved, the practitioner might move on to the neck and so on until the whole body has been assessed. This process normally takes several minutes per area, and is a very relaxed and un-rushed practice.

Another idea to consider when massaging is the use of symbols as aids in therapy. It is common for practitioners to incorporate symbols into their treatments. An appropriate symbol is normally drawn onto the body of the client at the beginning of a massage or the beginning of each different area in the treatment. This serves as an indicator and reminder to the practitioner and to the client that Reiki massage therapy has started or that a problem in an area has been resolved and treatment has moved to another area of the body. Sessions may also be conducted in a more specific way with the use of symbols if there is a definite issue that the client has. This might consist of the emotional symbol being used and meditated upon throughout the massage session if the client is having emotional issues of some description.

The fifth idea that may be included in Reiki energy massage therapy is the Kenyoku-ho brushing and bathing method. It is common for people practicing Reiki massages to use the brushing technique throughout the treatment at various stages. This may be pre-determined and specific or spontaneous dependent on the preference or schooling of the practitioner. Brushing here is used to disperse negative energy from the client throughout the session that may have accumulated during the therapy. Typical brushing techniques consist of brushing the energy diagonally from the body or brushing the negative energy off the client's arms or legs.

Another concept that is extremely important in Reiki massage treatments is the idea of self-treatment. A Reiki practitioner should always treat themselves and resolve any spiritual problems prior to carrying out a Reiki massage on somebody else so that their energies are harmonious and unobtrusive to the client. Something to consider for people interested in Reiki is that it is even possible to treat oneself and is not always necessary to see another practitioner about a problem that is manifesting. Many of these massage techniques that have been discussed in this chapter can be carried out in a personal way. For example, we can self-heal by touch in the same way that a practitioner might to others. starting at the head; unraveling and dealing with stress in that area before moving down the body as highlighted earlier in this chapter.

Using Reiki for disease or dis-ease is an idea familiar to most people who are interested in Reiki. It is common for specific ailments and issues to be identified or examined during a Reiki massage treatment. This is usually done by Byosen scanning. This technique is often integrated into Reiki massage treatments either as a type of checkup for the body or as an initial examination to see where there might be problem areas that need to be assessed.

The eighth idea to be considered in relation to Reiki massage treatment for beginners however is one that might not be so obvious to the reader. The idea of using Reiki treatment for pets is one that is often overlooked. Reiki can be used to help any living organism; namely anything with energy, a life force, spirit or soul. Animals can be treated in exactly the same way as humans by scanning and touching gently. The temperament of the animal might need to be considered however and some Reiki massage practices might not be appropriate for specific animals. Animals should be treated in the same way as humans are treated in Reiki sessions. Animals should always be given respect. The practitioner should always ask permission and only continue with treatment while the animal is content.

Reiki is now being practiced in conjunction with traditional massage therapy. Massage therapists are often trained in both traditional massage therapy as well as Reiki. Practitioners find it useful to administer Reiki to deal with the energy from a client after the regular massage. This combination of practices is becoming more popular in the modern era. It is not however practiced or even accepted by many Reiki practitioners. One of the potential issues with this modern hybrid is that the two practices are often confused with one another. It is important that the distinction is made between Reiki energy massage treatment and regular massage therapy. There is a danger that Reiki clients might expect a regular massage from a Reiki practitioner. Many Reiki practitioners also have an issue with combining the two practices because in many ways regular massage therapy and Reiki are opposing ideals. Reiki, as mentioned earlier, is unobtrusive, passive and is administered fully clothed. Traditional massage therapy is much more physical and forceful, a fact that many Reiki practitioners are against. It is purely dependent on the preferences of the individual.

The tenth idea to discuss in relation to Reiki is the traditional Japanese school of Reiki versus the more modern Western school. There is again some controversy among practitioners as some people feel the Japanese school is the true one and needs to be preserved and practiced. There are others who feel that the art of Reiki needs to evolve or else it will decline. There are also others who combine the two schools to suit their own preferences and style. There are some factors when practicing Reiki that are typically used by the original school such as the use of humming, chanting and a more prominent use of symbols. The western school however is more organized with specific practices and patterns being designed and followed by practitioners in a more standard format rather than treatment being unique for each client and individual. The school that each practitioner adopts, or specific elements from each school that are adopted is again entirely down to the individual.

A final idea to bear in mind when discussing Reiki massage therapy is to be open minded. Treatment must be carried out with the best intentions of the client at heart. If the client is not enjoying the therapy or an element of the therapy then a different technique or idea might be more appropriate. It is a good idea to allow the client to guide the therapy in a direction that they are comfortable. Reiki should be carried out on a mutually respectful basis. No treatment should ever be carried out without the complete comfort and approval of the client. It is beneficial therefore for the practitioner to enter into the therapy without expectation and to let the treatment unravel in a way that most suits the client.

Reflection & Summary

The aim of this book was to be an introduction to the practice of Reiki. The goal was to highlight how Reiki can be used by anybody. Reiki is not something that only Buddhists in far off lands wearing billowing robes partake in. Reiki is for everybody. It can enrich the lives of anyone who is willing to accept its power and undertake in its practice. This book was written as a tool to show everybody just how accessible it is. It was also written as an introduction and a foundation to Reiki, so that an interest in the magic of Reiki may be ignited in the reader that they might further their studies in Reiki. It is the hope that anybody reading this could one day study to be a Reiki master or teacher.

The entire concept of Reiki is that it is all inclusive. Everybody is joined by energy. Everybody exists because of energy. So much of Reiki is celebrating the universal connection that every living thing has through energy. It is allowing energy to flow through the body and from one organism to another in as harmonious a way as possible. Reiki is life.

Harnessing the power of energy is the most powerful tool a man has. By unlocking the power of the universe, he can reach his fullest potential and move past any obstacle it has. This power is a part of everything, so it can influence everything.

Having the ability to harness inner healing power can be used not for destructive means, but for the ability to heal yourself and others. Healing is the most powerful blessing we can give to one another. When we heal others, we are also healing ourselves and creating a better world. By learning to harness this energy to help others, we can learn to better ourselves and the lives of other people. Healing somebody is the most powerful gift we can give.

In this book all of the main introductory ideals of Reiki were covered. In chapter one a definition of Reiki was established. The nature of Reiki and the practices associated with it were discussed. The foundation of Reiki and the origin of the name were talked about. The essence of Reiki was realized. The fact that Reiki is spiritual but not necessarily religious was highlighted. Ambiguities surrounding Reiki were resolved. We discussed what Reiki actually is, not what it is perceived to be or pretends to be.

Chapter two talked about the benefits of Reiki. So many people wouldn't be aware of the sheer amount a human can gain from Reiki. Reiki can heal people physically, psychologically and spiritually. Reiki can relax, focus, enhance and benefit every time it is drawn upon. Reiki reduces stress and speeds up recovery. Reiki builds harmony and appreciation for everything.

In chapter three the Reiki symbols were discussed. Common uses of symbols were talked about. It was mentioned how symbols have been passed down from master to master, and how only second level practitioners or masters use symbols. It was emphasized that correct use of symbols during Reiki can greatly enhance the Reiki experience. Different uses of the symbols were then examined. Finally the five different symbols were talked about as well as the names and uses for all of them.

Chapter five was dedicated to the three pillars of Reiki. The three pillars were defined and the reasons for using the three pillars were discussed. It was mentioned how a Reiki healing session is possible without the three pillars but how the session is much more powerful when the healer prepares using the three pillars prior to healing. The purpose of each pillar was examined, firstly Gassho then Raiji-ho followed by Chiryo and the purpose of each pillar was discussed. It was also mentioned how Dr. Usui strongly advocated how important the use of the pillars was before a healing session. Reiki healing can be performed by first embracing the three pillars of Reiki, however, the powerful intention gained by first preparing and centering yourself in order to heal using Reiki spiritual energy will significantly enhance the effects of any Reiki healing session.

In chapter six some of the main Reiki techniques were introduced and talked about. This examined the three pillars also as techniques in Reiki. Techniques such as dry-bathing and scanning were talked about. It was mentioned how some of the more basic techniques such as Gassho were used in more complicated techniques such as Hatsurei-ho. It was also mentioned how Hatsurei-ho was one of the staple techniques of Reiki and how it is a foundation for all Reiki practice.

Finally in chapter seven some basic massage ideas for beginners were highlighted and suggested. These consisted of the healing touch and an examination of the chakras for use in massage therapy. Music was introduced as a useful tool for creating an atmosphere. The differences between a traditional massage and a Reiki energy massage were highlighted, and it was discussed how the two practices can work in tandem but how lots of Reiki practitioners are against this. This chapter ended with a brief discussion about the different Reiki schools from the Japanese and western traditions and the various features associated with each school.

This book covers all the basics of Reiki and will hopefully serve to help people develop an interest in it and become involved in the practice of Reiki. The goal of this book is to help people. There are so many people who suffer unnecessarily in this world and if the healing power of Reiki is spread throughout this planet more and more people will find the peace and joy that accompanies the practice of Reiki. If this book helped to reach just a few more people through you and bring them to happiness its goal was achieved.

THE END

"MEDITATION: THE PATH TO TRANQUILITY"
by Dominique Atkinson

What is Meditation?

The word meditation comes from two Latin words: Meditari, which means to think or exercise the mind and Mederi, which means to heal. It is interesting to note that the Sanskrit word Medha means wisdom.

Meditation can also be thought of as a stilling of the mind or thought processes. It is a state of consciousness where the mind is free from the random, scattered thoughts that have a way of intruding on us.

Classic yoga teaches that to reach the state of true meditation, a person must pass through several stages. Once the often complex rules of personal code, physical position, proper breathing and relaxation were attained, the person could move on to the more advanced practices of concentration, contemplation, and finally absorption.

There are an endless number of meditation variations in the world, but they all have a common goal – to allow people to calm their minds so that their baser instincts (cravings, impulses and harmful emotions) no longer distract or cause the person to act in a way that is not healthy. Through meditation anyone can learn to cultivate clarity, calmness, peace and well-being.

Modern meditation can refer to any one of these stages and different schools of yoga teach different methods. Some schools teach just relaxation, some focus on concentration techniques, and some teach a very relaxed and informal meditation that seems to have no ties to its eastern origins.

By regularly practicing a series of meditative techniques, it is possible to release the energy of the body and the mind, expanding the consciousness of practitioners.

While meditation seems to have eastern origins, many different religious traditions around the world practice one form of meditation or another. In fact, meditation does not need to be linked to any spiritual or religious path at all.

In the past thirty years, meditation has been embraced by many western practitioners with widely different spiritual beliefs. The physical, psychological and emotional benefits of meditation help ameliorate the stress inherent in the fast-paced western lifestyle. Meditation, quite simply, slows people down for a short time and gives them a breather.

Listening to music, contemplating a complex idea or taking a walk through the forest can all be meditative experiences. While they may not be considered meditation by hardcore yoga and meditation practitioners, anything that calms your mind and helps restore you balance is good, no matter what other people call it.

Meditation can be anything that stills your mind, provides you with a peaceful tranquility, eliminates your conscious thoughts and allows you to be present in the moment. There are two major categories that meditation practices fall into, concentrative and mindfulness.

Concentrative Meditation

Concentrative meditation teaches the student to focus on an image, the breath or a sound to calm the mind and allow a greater clarity and awareness to emerge. The most basic form of concentrative meditation is sitting still and focusing on the breath. When a person is under stress, the breathing becomes shallow and rapid. This leads to a very minor lack of oxygen, which in turn places the body under more stress. Focusing on deep, even breath breaks this cycle of emotional and physical stress and allows the person to begin to relax. Our bodies know this, and this is why when a person is upset we tell them to slow down and take a deep breath. We are encouraging the upset person to take a mini-meditative break.

Mindfulness Meditation

The purpose of mindfulness meditation is to allow practitioners to become more aware of the sensations and feelings around them, but as a passive observer, not a person who is reacting to them all. While practicing mindfulness meditation, the person will experience every part of their environment without conscious thought or reaction. He or she will sit quietly and notice everything that passes through the mind without reacting. This provides a sense of calm clarity.

Throughout this book we will discuss different meditation techniques and how to choose the one right for you. There is a technique for everyone and once you find the clarity and balance meditation has to offer, you will wonder how you ever did without it.

The Benefits of Meditation

When a person meditates, the body undergoes a series of physical changes that reduce stress and depression. This chapter lists many studies and results that link meditation to greater emotional, mental and physical health.

On the physical level, meditation has the following effects:

- Lowers blood pressure to a more normal level
- Decreases tension-related pain including headache, muscle tightness and ulcers
- Lessens insomnia
- Lowers the level of lactic acid in the blood which reduces physical anxiety
- Increases serotonin, which improves mood
- Strengthens the immune system
- Increases energy

On the mental level, meditation allows the brain to use an alpha brainwave pattern, allowing relaxation and healing. The effects include:

- ❖ Decreased anxiety
- ❖ Increased emotional stability
- ❖ Increased happiness
- ❖ Increased creativity
- ❖ Clarity
- ❖ Peace of mind
- ❖ Problems appear more manageable
- ❖ Sharpens thought

The Emotional Benefits of Meditation

There is no disputing the fact that meditation provides strong, long-lasting benefits for the mental and emotional states of its practitioners. The regular practice of meditation enhances a positive outlook on life and a positive self-image.

Meditation Regulates Mood and Anxiety Disorders

An analysis of over 20 studies focusing on meditation and yoga published in PubMed and PsychInfo concluded that meditation can treat anxiety as well as antidepressant therapy. If you are taking antidepressant medication, do not stop taking it when you begin meditation. Allow the meditation process to take root and then speak to your physician before making any changes in your medication.

Meditation Calms Mothers-to-Be

Pregnant women at risk for or already suffering from depression that took part in a ten week mindfulness and yoga training program reported reduced symptoms of depression. They also showed stronger bonding with their babies before birth.

Meditation Reduces General Anxiety and Stress

Open Monitoring Meditation, the practice of being aware of thoughts without acting on them, reduces the density of grey matter in the stress and anxiety related areas of the brain. Participants in a study from the University of Wisconsin-Madison reported an increased ability to focus on their current surroundings without becoming upset over any particular thing. The ability to allow things to pass without strong reaction reduces anxiety and stress.

Meditation Reduces Symptoms of Panic Disorder

A paper in the American Journal of Psychiatry reported that after three months of meditation training, 20 of 22 patients showed substantial decreases in the effects of panic and anxiety. When followed up at a later date, those benefits were still being felt.

Meditation Increases Brain Growth

Harvard neuroscientists studied 16 people during and after an 8 week mindfulness course. Participants used guided meditation and incorporated mindfulness throughout their daily activities. At the end of the study, MRI scans showed an increase in the gray matter in areas of the brain that dealt with memory, self-image, and regulation of emotion and sense of perspective.

Other studies have shown increases in the hippocampus and frontal lobes.

Meditation may Decrease Sleep Requirements
Research conducted by the University of Kentucky showed that even novice meditators required fewer hours of sleep per night after meditating. The difference was more striking with experienced meditators. Meditation cannot replace all your sleep needs, but it can give you a boost if you need it

Meditation Helps Control Substance Abuse
Three studies using mindfulness meditation and incarcerated participants show a link between meditation and lowered substance abuse.

The Mental Benefits of Meditation
Simply put, meditation helps your brain work better. People who meditate on a regular basis report that they can concentrate more effectively and are able to work efficiently under stress.

Meditation Improves Focus and Attention
A University of California study shows that after meditation, participants were able to focus on dull and repetitive tasks more effectively.

With 20 minutes of meditation per day, students increased their cognitive skills by up to ten times. They were also able to perform better on stress-inducing timed tests.

Meditation helps to thicken the prefrontal cortex and can help stave off the loss of cognitive ability associated with old age.

Meditation Improves Information Processing
Long-term meditation practitioners show increased folding, or gyrification, of the cortex which indicates the brain has an increased ability to process information, and to process it faster. This allows people to make good decisions faster, form stronger memories and benefit from an increased attention span.

Meditation Decreases the Sensation of Pain
Researchers at the University of Montreal studied 26 participants, 13 Zen masters and 13 non-meditators. They exposed the participants to the same amount of pain-inducing heat and measured brain activity with an fMRI scanner. The Zen masters reported less pain, and their fMRI scans confirmed that they actually felt less pain.

In fact, in another study at the Wake Forest Baptist Medical Center meditation was shown to be more effective than morphine for pain control. After an hour of meditation training, participants reported a 40 percent reduction in pain intensity and a 57 percent reduction in the unpleasantness of pain. Morphine or other pain-relieving drugs typically reduce pain ratings by 25 percent.

Meditation Helps Manage ADHD
A study of 50 adult ADHD patients who had undergone mindfulness meditation training showed reduced hyperactivity, reduced impulsivity and an increased ability to act with awareness. This combination led to an overall improvement in ADHD symptoms.

Meditation Increases Focus, Even in Distracting Environments
Emory University researchers showed that participants in a study who had previously been trained in meditation showed increased connectivity in the attention-controlling areas of the brain. This helped the participants keep their focus and ignore distractions, even at times when they were not meditating.

Meditation Keeps You from Multitasking
Multitasking is a productivity myth. You may feel as though you are getting more work done but you aren't. Multitasking splits your attention and causes stress.

When a person attempts to multitask, they wind up feeling distracted and stressed. Research conducted at the University of Washington and the University of Arizona with human resources personnel showed that those who practiced meditation reported lower levels of stress and had better memory when tested. They were able to focus on tasks for longer periods of time, decreasing the overall amount of time necessary for task completion.

Meditation Helps Allocate Brain Resources
When the brain is given two almost simultaneous tasks to concentrate on, the second is often unintentionally ignored. This effect is called attention blink. Research participants who spent three months of mindfulness meditation were able to decrease or eliminate their 'attention blink', allowing them to recognize both tasks. This shows less allocation of brain resources for each task, meaning they required less attention to focus and remember each task, not that they used less brain power to work on each task.

Meditation Improves Visual and Spatial Processing
With one to four sessions of mindfulness meditation training, working memory, executive function and visuospatial processing increased

Mindfulness Meditation Enhances Creativity
Research from Leiden University in The Netherlands showed that open monitoring meditation enhances creativity and the ability to think along new paths. Participants who participated in open monitoring meditation performed better than those who did not meditate when asked to develop new ideas.

Meditation and the Body
With all the benefits meditation provides for the brain and emotions, it is no surprise that meditation also benefits the physical body.

Meditation reduces the risk of heart disease and stroke
Heart disease is the largest killer in the world. In a 2012 study, 200 high-risk participants were asked to take either a transcendental meditation class or a health education class geared toward a healthy diet and exercise routine. Over the next five years, researchers found that the participants who chose the transcendental meditation course had a 48 percent decrease in their risk of heart attack, stroke or death.

The study noted that meditation "significantly reduced risk for mortality, myocardial infarction, and stroke in coronary heart disease patients. These changes were associated with lower blood pressure and psychosocial stress factors."

Meditation affects the expression of Stress and Immunity Genes
Harvard Medical School studies show that after practicing meditation and yoga, participants showed increased mitochondrial energy production, consumption and resiliency. This in turn provided the participants with higher immunity and resilience to stress.

Meditation Reduces Blood Pressure
Relaxation allows for the formation of nitric oxide, which opens the blood vessels. Research has shown that Zen meditation reduces blood pressure. Relaxation response meditation has shown 2/3 of participants with lowered blood pressure after three months. This resulted in them requiring less medication.

Mindfulness and Inflammatory Disorders
Mindfulness meditation produces a wide variety of effects of patients, including reduced levels of pro-inflammatory genes, allowing participants to physically recover from a stress-inducing situation more quickly.

Meditation Helps You Live Longer
Data suggest that some forms of meditation helps stave off the shortening of telomeres (this is the basis of the aging process) by reducing stress arousal, cognitive stress and increasing positive states of mind and hormonal production.

Meditation and Personal Relationships
Now that meditation has helped our minds, emotions and bodies we are feeling quite good. It's no wonder that our interpersonal relationships will also improve.

Meditation Improves Empathy
The Buddhist practice of metta, or loving-kindness meditation, boosts people's ability to read facial expressions and empathize with others. Developing compassion increases the loving attitude one has for others, self-acceptance, social support and a general feeling of competence.

Metta Reduces Feelings of Social Isolation

A study published by the American Psychological Association reports that when participants spent just a few minutes in Metta meditation, they had increased feelings of positivity toward strangers, more feelings of social connection. This easily implemented technique increases positive social emotions and decreases feelings of isolation, even when people are still actually alone.

Science confirms the benefits practitioners of meditation have been espousing for centuries: Meditation promotes good health, prevents diseases, increases happiness, focuses concentration and allows you to feel more harmony throughout the world...

[Excerpts from the first 3 Chapters – for complete book, please purchase on Amazon.com]